Almond Flour Recipes

A Beginner's Guide to Getting Started, With Over 50 Gluten-Free Recipes

copyright © 2024 Bruce Ackerberg

All rights reserved No part of this book may be reproduced, or stored in a retrieval system, or transmitted in any form or by any means, electronic, mechanical, photocopying, recording, or otherwise, without express written permission of the publisher.

Disclaimer

By reading this disclaimer, you are accepting the terms of the disclaimer in full. If you disagree with this disclaimer, please do not read the guide.

All of the content within this guide is provided for informational and educational purposes only, and should not be accepted as independent medical or other professional advice. The author is not a doctor, physician, nurse, mental health provider, or registered nutritionist/dietician. Therefore, using and reading this guide does not establish any form of a physician-patient relationship.

Always consult with a physician or another qualified health provider with any issues or questions you might have regarding any sort of medical condition. Do not ever disregard any qualified professional medical advice or delay seeking that advice because of anything you have read in this guide. The information in this guide is not intended to be any sort of medical advice and should not be used in lieu of any medical advice by a licensed and qualified medical professional.

The information in this guide has been compiled from a variety of known sources. However, the author cannot attest to or guarantee the accuracy of each source and thus should not be held liable for any errors or omissions.

You acknowledge that the publisher of this guide will not be held liable for any loss or damage of any kind incurred as a result of this guide or the reliance on any information provided within this guide. You acknowledge and agree that you assume all risk and responsibility for any action you undertake in response to the information in this guide.

Using this guide does not guarantee any particular result (e.g., weight loss or a cure). By reading this guide, you acknowledge that there are no guarantees to any specific outcome or results you can expect.

All product names, diet plans, or names used in this guide are for identification purposes only and are the property of their respective owners. The use of these names does not imply endorsement. All other trademarks cited herein are the property of their respective owners.

Where applicable, this guide is not intended to be a substitute for the original work of this diet plan and is, at most, a supplement to the original work for this diet plan and never a direct substitute. This guide is a personal expression of the facts of that diet plan.

Where applicable, persons shown in the cover images are stock photography models and the publisher has obtained the rights to use the images through license agreements with third-party stock image companies.

Table of Contents

Introduction	**8**
Everything You Need to Know About Almond Flour	**10**
Types of Almond Flour: Blanched vs. Unblanched	10
Common Uses in Cooking and Baking	11
History of Almond Cultivation	**13**
The Development of Almond Flour Production	14
Production Process from Almond to Flour	14
Health Benefits of Almond Flour	**16**
Nutritional Profile of Almond Flour	16
Benefits for Specific Diets	18
Impact on Blood Sugar Levels	19
Benefits of Heart Health	19
Influence on Gut Health and Digestion	20
Potential Allergenic Considerations	21
Sample Recipes	**22**
Almond Flour Pancakes	23
Almond Flour Muffins	24
Almond Flour Waffles	25
Almond Flour Smoothie Bowls	26
Almond Flour Breakfast Bars	27
Almond Flour Quiche	28
Almond Flour Biscuits	30
Almond Flour Granola	31
Almond Flour Crepes	32
Almond Flour Bagels	33
Almond Flour Bread for Sandwiches	35
Almond Flour Pizza Crust	37
Almond Flour Tortillas	38
Almond Flour Breadsticks	39

Almond Flour Crab Cakes	40
Almond Flour Chicken Tenders	41
Almond Flour Veggie Patties	42
Almond Flour Flatbreads	43
Almond Flour Pasta	44
Almond Flour Soup Thickener	45
Almond-Crusted Salmon	46
Almond Flour Meatballs	47
Almond Flour Lasagna	49
Almond Flour Battered Fish	51
Almond Flour Stuffed Peppers	52
Almond Flour Chicken Parmesan	54
Almond Flour Zucchini Fries	56
Almond Flour Meatloaf	57
Almond Flour Cauliflower Pizza	58
Almond Flour Gnocchi	60
Almond Flour Chocolate Chip Cookies	61
Almond Flour Brownies	63
Almond Flour Cupcakes	64
Almond Flour Cheesecake Crust	65
Almond Flour Banana Bread	66
Almond Flour Macaroons	67
Almond Flour Donuts	68
Almond Flour Scones	69
Almond Flour Crackers	71
Almond Flour Energy Balls	73
Almond Flour Pretzels	74
Almond Flour Granola Bars	75
Almond Flour Cheese Straws	76
Almond Flour Protein Bites	77
Almond Flour Popcorn Chicken	78

Almond Flour Onion Rings	79
Almond Flour Crisps	80
Almond Flour Fruit Tarts	81

6 Step-by-Step Plan to Start Incorporating Almond Flour into Your Recipes — **83**

Step 1: Choose the Right Almond Flour	83
Step 2: Understand its Properties	85
Step 3: Start with Simple Recipes	87
Step 4: Substitute Almond Flour in Traditional Recipes	88
Step 5: Appreciate the Benefits	91
Step 6: Experiment and Innovate	92

Conclusion — **97**

FAQs — **100**

References and Helpful Links — **103**

Introduction

As more people become health-conscious and seek alternatives to traditional wheat flour, almond flour has emerged as a popular choice for those looking to enhance their diets. This versatile and nutritious ingredient, made from finely ground blanched or unblanched almonds, offers a wealth of health benefits and can be used in a wide array of recipes, from breakfast to dessert.

In today's modern diets, almond flour is celebrated not only for its rich, nutty flavor but also for its impressive nutritional profile. Packed with protein, healthy fats, fiber, and essential vitamins and minerals, it is a fantastic option for individuals following gluten-free, paleo, or keto diets. Moreover, its low carbohydrate content makes it an excellent choice for those looking to maintain stable blood sugar levels.

In this guide, we will talk about the following:

- Everything You Need to Know About Almond Flour
- History of Almond Cultivation
- Health Benefits of Almond Flour
- Sample Recipes

- Step-by-Step Plan to Start Incorporating Almond Flour into Your Recipes

Almond flour's growing popularity is also a testament to its adaptability across various cuisines, contributing to culinary innovation and supporting sustainable agriculture. Its appeal transcends diverse dietary preferences, making it a key ingredient in the quest for healthier, more sustainable eating habits. By the end of this guide, you will have a comprehensive understanding of almond flour and how to incorporate it into your diet for maximum health benefits.

Everything You Need to Know About Almond Flour

Almond flour is a finely ground flour made from whole almonds. Typically, almonds are blanched to remove their skins and then ground to produce a fine, powdery texture. This flour retains all the nutritional benefits of almonds, making it a popular alternative to traditional wheat flour. Known for its slightly sweet and nutty flavor, almond flour is an excellent ingredient for a variety of culinary applications.

Types of Almond Flour: Blanched vs. Unblanched

Almond flour comes in two main types: blanched and unblanched. The key difference between them lies in whether the almond skins are removed before grinding.

- *Blanched Almond Flour*: This type is made from almonds that have had their skins removed through a blanching process. The almonds are briefly boiled and cooled, and then their skins are peeled off before being ground into flour. Blanched almond flour is lighter in color and finer in texture, making it ideal for recipes where a smooth texture is desired, such as cakes, cookies, and pastries.

- ***Unblanched Almond Flour***: Unlike blanched almond flour, unblanched almond flour is made from almonds that still have their skins on. This results in a coarser texture and a slightly darker color due to the presence of the almond skins. Unblanched almond flour is often used in recipes where a more robust texture is acceptable or even desirable, such as in bread, muffins, and some savory dishes.

Common Uses in Cooking and Baking

Almond flour's versatility makes it a favorite among both amateur and professional chefs. Here are some of the most common uses of almond flour in cooking and baking:

- ***Baking***: Almond flour can be used to create a variety of baked goods, including cakes, cookies, muffins, and bread. Its fine texture and nutty flavor enhance the taste and nutritional profile of these treats.
- ***Gluten-Free Recipes***: Since almond flour is naturally gluten-free, it's a go-to ingredient for those with gluten sensitivities or celiac disease. It can replace wheat flour in many recipes, providing a similar structure and consistency.

- ***Low-Carb and Keto Diets***: Almond flour is low in carbohydrates and high in healthy fats, making it an excellent choice for those following low-carb or ketogenic diets. It's often used to make low-carb versions of traditional high-carb dishes like pizza crust, pancakes, and bread.
- ***Thickening Agent***: In sauces and gravies, almond flour can be used as a thickening agent, adding both body and flavor.
- ***Breadcrumb Substitute***: Almond flour can be used in place of breadcrumbs for coating meats or vegetables before frying or baking, giving dishes a crispy, flavorful crust.
- ***Pasta and Noodles***: It can also be used to make gluten-free pasta and noodles, offering a nutritious alternative to traditional pasta.

Almond flour's growing popularity is a testament to its adaptability and the myriad of health benefits it offers. Whether you're baking a batch of cookies, making a savory quiche, or thickening a creamy sauce, almond flour is a versatile ingredient that can elevate your dishes while keeping them nutritious and delicious.

History of Almond Cultivation

Almonds have been cultivated for thousands of years, with their origins tracing back to the Middle East. Historical evidence suggests that almond trees were among the first domesticated fruit trees, with cultivation dating back to around 3000 B.C. The ancient civilizations of Mesopotamia and Egypt prized almonds for their nutritional value and versatility. Almonds were even found in the tomb of Tutankhamun, highlighting their importance in ancient diets and cultures.

As trade routes expanded, almonds spread throughout the Mediterranean region. The Greeks and Romans played significant roles in popularizing almonds across Europe. By the Middle Ages, almonds had become a staple in European cuisine, commonly used in both savory and sweet dishes. The almond's journey continued as explorers and settlers introduced it to the New World, particularly in California, which would eventually become a global leader in almond production.

The Development of Almond Flour Production

The production of almond flour has evolved significantly over the centuries. Initially, almond flour was made by manually grinding almonds using stones or primitive mills. This labor-intensive process limited its availability and use. However, as milling technology advanced, so did the efficiency of almond flour production.

In the 20th century, industrial milling techniques revolutionized the production of almond flour. Automated blanching and grinding processes allowed for the mass production of both blanched and unblanched almond flour. This increased accessibility and affordability, making almond flour a common ingredient in households and commercial kitchens alike. The rise of gluten-free and low-carb diets in recent years has further boosted the popularity of almond flour, leading to innovations in its production and applications.

Production Process from Almond to Flour

The production of almond flour involves several key steps, ensuring the final product is of high quality and retains its nutritional benefits:

1. *Harvesting*: Almonds are typically harvested from late August to October. The trees are shaken to release the almonds, which are then collected from the ground.

2. ***Blanching (for Blanched Almond Flour)***: The almonds are briefly boiled to soften their skins. After cooling, the skins are removed, leaving behind the white, blanched almonds.
3. ***Drying***: The blanched or unblanched almonds are dried to remove excess moisture. This step is crucial to achieve the desired texture and shelf life of the flour.
4. ***Grinding***: The almonds are ground into a fine powder using industrial mills. For blanched almond flour, the grinding process ensures a smooth, fine texture. Unblanched almond flour, which includes the almond skins, results in a coarser texture.
5. ***Sifting***: The ground almonds are sifted to remove any larger particles, ensuring a consistent and fine flour.
6. ***Packaging***: The almond flour is packaged in moisture-proof bags to maintain freshness and prevent contamination.

Overall, the production process of almond flour requires careful handling and processing to ensure a high-quality final product.

Health Benefits of Almond Flour

Almond flour is not only a versatile ingredient in the kitchen but also a nutritional powerhouse. Packed with essential macronutrients, vitamins, and minerals, it offers numerous health benefits. Suitable for gluten-free, paleo, and keto diets, almond flour supports various dietary needs. It helps manage blood sugar levels, promotes heart health, and aids in digestion. However, it's important to be mindful of potential allergenic considerations. In this chapter, we'll explore the specific health benefits of almond flour and how it can contribute to a balanced and healthy diet.

Nutritional Profile of Almond Flour

Almond flour is a nutritional powerhouse, packed with essential macronutrients, vitamins, and minerals that contribute to overall health and wellness.

1. **Macronutrients**
    - *Protein*: Almond flour is a good source of plant-based protein, providing about 6 grams

per quarter cup. Protein is essential for muscle repair, immune function, and overall growth.
- *Healthy Fats*: They contain a high amount of healthy fats, particularly monounsaturated fats, which are known to support heart health by reducing bad cholesterol levels.
- *Fiber*: Almond flour is rich in dietary fiber, offering about 3 grams per quarter cup. Fiber aids in digestion, helps maintain healthy blood sugar levels and keeps you feeling full longer.
- *Low Carbs*: With only about 6 grams of carbohydrates per quarter cup, almond flour is a low-carb alternative to traditional wheat flour, making it suitable for low-carb and ketogenic diets.

2. **Vitamins and Minerals**
   - *Vitamin E*: Almond flour is an excellent source of vitamin E, an antioxidant that helps protect your cells from oxidative damage. One serving can provide up to 35% of your daily recommended intake.
   - *Magnesium*: This mineral is crucial for muscle function, blood sugar regulation, and energy production. Almond flour contains a significant amount of magnesium, which supports these vital bodily functions.

- *Calcium*: Essential for bone health, calcium is found in almond flour in smaller amounts compared to dairy but still contributes to your daily intake.
- *Iron*: Almond flour provides iron, which is necessary for the production of red blood cells and the transportation of oxygen throughout the body.

Benefits for Specific Diets

Almond flour is versatile and fits well into various dietary plans, making it a preferred choice for many health-conscious individuals.

1. **Gluten-Free Diets**

   For those with gluten intolerance or celiac disease, almond flour is an excellent gluten-free alternative to wheat flour. It allows for the enjoyment of baked goods and other recipes without the adverse effects associated with gluten consumption.

2. **Paleo Diets**

   The paleo diet emphasizes whole, unprocessed foods that would have been available to our ancestors. Almond flour, being minimally processed and derived from a natural source, fits perfectly into this dietary plan.

3. **Keto Diets**

   The ketogenic diet focuses on low-carb, high-fat foods to induce ketosis. Almond flour's low carbohydrate content and high-fat profile make it a staple in keto-friendly recipes, allowing for the creation of delicious, compliant baked goods and meals.

Impact on Blood Sugar Levels

1. **Low Glycemic Index**

   Almond flour has a low glycemic index, which means it does not cause rapid spikes in blood sugar levels. This makes it an ideal choice for those managing diabetes or anyone looking to maintain stable energy levels throughout the day.

2. **Stabilizing Blood Sugar**

   The combination of fiber, protein, and healthy fats in almond flour helps to slow the absorption of sugar into the bloodstream, preventing sudden drops and spikes in blood sugar levels. This stabilizing effect can improve overall energy levels and reduce cravings.

Benefits of Heart Health

Almond flour supports heart health in several ways:

1. **Monounsaturated Fats**

   The high content of monounsaturated fats in almond flour helps to lower LDL (bad) cholesterol levels while maintaining or even raising HDL (good) cholesterol levels. This balance is crucial for reducing the risk of heart disease.

2. **Antioxidants and Vitamin E**

   Vitamin E acts as a potent antioxidant, protecting the heart and blood vessels from oxidative stress and inflammation. Regular consumption of almond flour can contribute to improved cardiovascular health.

Influence on Gut Health and Digestion

1. **Dietary Fiber**

   Fiber is essential for a healthy digestive system. The fiber in almond flour promotes regular bowel movements and helps prevent constipation. It also acts as a prebiotic, feeding the beneficial bacteria in your gut and supporting a balanced microbiome.

2. **Prebiotic Properties**

   The prebiotic properties of almond flour's fiber content help to nourish the gut microbiota, which plays a crucial role in digestion, immune function, and overall health. A healthy gut microbiome can enhance nutrient absorption and reduce inflammation.

Potential Allergenic Considerations

1. **Tree Nut Allergies and Symptoms**

   Almond flour is derived from almonds, a type of tree nut. Individuals with tree nut allergies should avoid almond flour to prevent allergic reactions. Common symptoms of a tree nut allergy include itching, swelling, difficulty breathing, and anaphylaxis, which is a severe, life-threatening reaction.

2. **Precautions and Alternatives**

   If you or someone you're serving has a tree nut allergy, it's important to take precautions. Alternatives to almond flour include coconut flour, sunflower seed flour, and oat flour, which can often be used in similar recipes with some adjustments.

Almond flour offers a strong nutritional profile and many health benefits, making it a great addition to a health-conscious diet. However, it's crucial to consider potential allergies and choose suitable alternatives when needed. By incorporating almond flour into your meals and snacks, you can enjoy its benefits while supporting your overall well-being.

Sample Recipes

In this chapter, we'll provide a few sample recipes to inspire you to start incorporating almond flour into your cooking. These recipes are simple, delicious, and packed with nutrients.

Breakfast Recipes Using Almond Flour

Almond Flour Pancakes

Ingredients:

- 1 cup almond flour
- 2 large eggs
- 1/4 cup unsweetened almond milk
- 1 tbsp honey or maple syrup
- 1 tsp vanilla extract
- 1/2 tsp baking powder
- Pinch of salt
- Butter or oil for cooking

Instructions:

1. In a mixing bowl, whisk together the eggs, almond milk, honey, and vanilla extract.
2. Add the almond flour, baking powder, and salt to the wet ingredients and stir until well combined.
3. Heat a non-stick skillet over medium heat and add a bit of butter or oil.
4. Pour 1/4 cup of batter onto the skillet and cook until bubbles form on the surface, then flip and cook until golden brown.
5. Serve warm with your favorite toppings.

Almond Flour Muffins

Ingredients:

- 2 cups almond flour
- 3 large eggs
- 1/4 cup honey or maple syrup
- 1/4 cup unsweetened almond milk
- 1 tsp vanilla extract
- 1 tsp baking soda
- Pinch of salt
- Optional: blueberries, chocolate chips, or nuts

Instructions:

1. Warm your oven to 350°F (175°C) and place paper liners in a muffin tin.
2. In a big bowl, beat together the eggs, honey, almond milk, and vanilla extract.
3. Add the almond flour, baking soda, and salt, and mix until smooth.
4. Fold in any optional add-ins like blueberries or chocolate chips.
5. Divide the batter evenly among the muffin cups.
6. Bake for 20-25 minutes, or until a toothpick inserted into the center comes out clean.
7. Allow to cool before serving.

Almond Flour Waffles

Ingredients:

- 1 1/2 cups almond flour
- 3 large eggs
- 1/4 cup unsweetened almond milk
- 2 tbsp melted coconut oil or butter
- 1 tbsp honey or maple syrup
- 1 tsp vanilla extract
- 1 tsp baking powder
- Pinch of salt

Instructions:

1. Preheat your waffle iron according to the manufacturer's instructions.
2. In a big bowl, mix the eggs, almond milk, melted coconut oil, honey, and vanilla extract together with a whisk.
3. Add the almond flour, baking powder, and salt to the wet ingredients and mix until smooth.
4. Grease the waffle iron with a bit of oil or cooking spray.
5. Pour the batter into the waffle iron and cook according to the manufacturer's instructions until golden brown.
6. Serve with your favorite toppings.

Almond Flour Smoothie Bowls

Ingredients:

- 1/2 cup almond flour
- 1 frozen banana
- 1/2 cup frozen berries
- 1/2 cup unsweetened almond milk
- 1 tbsp almond butter
- 1 tsp honey or maple syrup (optional)
- Toppings: fresh fruit, granola, nuts, seeds

Instructions:

1. In a blender, combine the frozen banana, frozen berries, almond milk, almond butter, and almond flour.
2. Blend until smooth and creamy. Add more almond milk if needed to reach the desired consistency.
3. Pour the smoothie into a bowl and top with your favorite toppings.
4. Serve immediately.

Almond Flour Breakfast Bars

Ingredients:

- 2 cups almond flour
- 1/2 cup unsweetened shredded coconut
- 1/4 cup honey or maple syrup
- 1/4 cup melted coconut oil
- 1 tsp vanilla extract
- 1/2 tsp baking soda
- Pinch of salt
- Optional: dried fruit, nuts, or chocolate chips

Instructions:

1. Set your oven to 350°F (175°C) and prepare an 8x8 inch baking dish by lining it with parchment paper.
2. Combine the almond flour, shredded coconut, honey, melted coconut oil, vanilla extract, baking soda, and salt in a big bowl.
3. Fold in any optional add-ins like dried fruit or nuts.
4. Press the mixture evenly into the prepared baking pan.
5. Bake for 20-25 minutes, or until golden brown.
6. Allow to cool completely before cutting into bars.

Almond Flour Quiche

Ingredients:

For the Crust:

- 1 1/2 cups almond flour
- 1/4 cup melted butter or coconut oil
- 1 large egg
- Pinch of salt

For the Filling:

- 4 large eggs
- 1/2 cup heavy cream or unsweetened almond milk
- 1 cup cooked vegetables (spinach, mushrooms, peppers, etc.)
- 1/2 cup shredded cheese (optional)
- Salt and pepper to taste

Instructions:

1. Set your oven to 350°F (175°C) and lightly coat a 9-inch pie dish with grease.
2. In a bowl, mix together the almond flour, melted butter, egg, and salt until a dough forms.
3. Press the dough evenly into the bottom and sides of the pie dish.
4. Bake the crust for 10 minutes, then remove from the oven.

5. In a separate bowl, whisk together the eggs, cream, cooked vegetables, cheese, salt, and pepper.
6. Pour the filling into the pre-baked crust.
7. Bake for 25-30 minutes, or until the filling is set and the top is golden brown.
8. Allow to cool slightly before slicing and serving.

Almond Flour Biscuits

Ingredients:

- 2 cups almond flour
- 1/4 cup melted butter or coconut oil
- 2 large eggs
- 1 tbsp honey or maple syrup
- 1 tsp baking powder
- 1/4 tsp salt

Instructions:

1. Warm up your oven to 350°F (175°C) and cover a baking sheet with parchment paper.
2. Combine almond flour, melted butter, eggs, honey, baking powder, and salt in a large bowl, stirring until a dough forms.
3. Scoop the dough onto the prepared baking sheet, forming biscuits.
4. Bake for 15-20 minutes or until golden brown.
5. Serve warm with butter or your favorite toppings.

Almond Flour Granola

Ingredients:

- 2 cups rolled oats
- 1 cup almond flour
- 1/2 cup chopped nuts (almonds, walnuts, etc.)
- 1/4 cup honey or maple syrup
- 1/4 cup melted coconut oil
- 1 tsp vanilla extract
- 1/2 tsp cinnamon
- Pinch of salt
- Optional: dried fruit, chocolate chips

Instructions:

1. Warm up your oven to 350°F (175°C) and cover a baking sheet with parchment paper.
2. Combine rolled oats, almond flour, chopped nuts, honey, melted coconut oil, vanilla extract, cinnamon, and salt in a large bowl, stirring well.
3. Spread the mixture evenly onto the prepared baking sheet.
4. Bake for 20-25 minutes, stirring halfway through, until golden brown.
5. Allow to cool completely, then stir in any optional add-ins like dried fruit or chocolate chips.
6. Store in an airtight container.

Almond Flour Crepes

Ingredients:

- 1 cup almond flour
- 3 large eggs
- 1/2 cup unsweetened almond milk
- 1 tbsp melted butter or coconut oil
- 1 tsp vanilla extract
- Pinch of salt

Instructions:

1. In a blender, combine the almond flour, eggs, almond milk, melted butter, vanilla extract, and salt. Blend until smooth.
2. Heat a non-stick skillet over medium heat and lightly grease with butter or oil.
3. Pour a small amount of batter into the skillet, swirling to coat the bottom evenly.
4. Cook until the edges begin to lift and the crepe is lightly browned, then flip and cook the other side.
5. Repeat with the remaining batter.
6. Fill with your favorite sweet or savory fillings and serve.

Almond Flour Bagels

Ingredients:

- 2 cups almond flour
- 1/4 cup coconut flour
- 1/4 cup psyllium husk powder
- 1 tbsp baking powder
- 1/2 tsp salt
- 1 cup boiling water
- 2 large eggs, beaten
- 2 tbsp apple cider vinegar
- Optional toppings: sesame seeds, poppy seeds, everything bagel seasoning

Instructions:

1. Warm up your oven to 350°F (175°C) and cover a baking sheet with parchment paper.
2. In a large mixing bowl, blend together almond flour, coconut flour, psyllium husk powder, baking powder, and salt.
3. Pour the boiling water into the dry ingredients and stir quickly until well combined.
4. Add the beaten eggs and apple cider vinegar to the mixture, continuing to stir until a dough forms.
5. Divide the dough into 6 equal portions and roll each portion into a ball.

6. Flatten each ball slightly and use your finger to create a hole in the center, forming a bagel shape.
7. Place the bagels on the prepared baking sheet and sprinkle with optional toppings if desired.
8. Bake for 25-30 minutes, or until the bagels are golden brown and firm to the touch.
9. Allow to cool on a wire rack before serving.

Lunch Recipes Using Almond Flour

Almond Flour Bread for Sandwiches

Ingredients:

- 2 cups almond flour
- 1/4 cup coconut flour
- 1/4 cup psyllium husk powder
- 1 tbsp baking powder
- 1/2 tsp salt
- 4 large eggs
- 1/4 cup melted butter or coconut oil
- 1 cup unsweetened almond milk
- 1 tbsp apple cider vinegar

Instructions:

1. Warm up your oven to 350°F (175°C) and cover a baking sheet with parchment paper.
2. In a big mixing bowl, stir together the almond flour, coconut flour, psyllium husk powder, baking powder, and salt.
3. In another bowl, whisk together the eggs, melted butter, almond milk, and apple cider vinegar.
4. Pour the wet ingredients into the dry ingredients and stir until well combined.

5. Pour the batter into the prepared loaf pan and smooth the top.
6. Bake for 50-60 minutes, or until a toothpick inserted into the center comes out clean.
7. Allow the bread to cool completely before slicing and serving.

Almond Flour Pizza Crust

Ingredients:

- 2 cups almond flour
- 2 large eggs
- 1/4 cup grated parmesan cheese
- 1 tbsp olive oil
- 1 tsp baking powder
- 1/2 tsp salt
- 1/2 tsp garlic powder
- 1/2 tsp dried oregano

Instructions:

1. Heat your oven to 375°F (190°C) and place parchment paper on a baking sheet.
2. In a sizable bowl, combine almond flour, eggs, parmesan cheese, olive oil, baking powder, salt, garlic powder, and dried oregano until a dough forms.
3. Place the dough on the prepared baking sheet and press it into a thin, even circle or rectangle.
4. Bake for 15-20 minutes, or until the edges are golden brown.
5. Remove from the oven, add your favorite pizza toppings, and return to the oven for an additional 10-15 minutes, or until the toppings are cooked to your liking.
6. Slice and serve.

Almond Flour Tortillas

Ingredients:

- 2 cups almond flour
- 2 large eggs
- 1/4 cup water
- 1 tbsp olive oil
- 1/2 tsp salt

Instructions:

1. In a big bowl, blend the almond flour, eggs, water, olive oil, and salt until the dough takes shape.
2. Divide the dough into 6 equal portions and roll each portion into a ball.
3. Place each ball between two sheets of parchment paper and roll it out into a thin circle.
4. Heat a non-stick skillet over medium heat and cook each tortilla for 1-2 minutes on each side, or until lightly browned and cooked through.
5. Serve warm with your favorite fillings.

Almond Flour Breadsticks

Ingredients:

- 2 cups almond flour
- 1/4 cup grated parmesan cheese
- 2 large eggs
- 1 tbsp olive oil
- 1 tsp baking powder
- 1/2 tsp garlic powder
- 1/2 tsp dried oregano
- 1/2 tsp salt

Instructions:

1. Warm up your oven to 350°F (175°C) and cover a baking sheet with parchment paper.
2. In a sizable bowl, blend the almond flour, parmesan cheese, eggs, olive oil, baking powder, garlic powder, dried oregano, and salt until the dough takes shape.
3. Roll the dough into long, thin sticks and place them on the prepared baking sheet.
4. Bake for 15-20 minutes or until golden brown and crispy.
5. Serve warm with your favorite dipping sauce.

Almond Flour Crab Cakes

Ingredients:

- 1 lb crab meat
- 1/2 cup almond flour
- 1/4 cup mayonnaise
- 1 large egg
- 1 tbsp Dijon mustard
- 1 tbsp lemon juice
- 1 tsp Old Bay seasoning
- 1/4 tsp salt
- 1/4 tsp black pepper
- 2 tbsp olive oil for frying

Instructions:

1. In a sizable bowl, mix the crab meat, almond flour, mayonnaise, egg, Dijon mustard, lemon juice, Old Bay seasoning, salt, and black pepper together.
2. Form the mixture into 8 patties.
3. Heat the olive oil in a large skillet over medium heat.
4. Cook the crab cakes for 3-4 minutes on each side, or until golden brown and crispy.
5. Serve warm with tartar sauce or your favorite dipping sauce.

Almond Flour Chicken Tenders

Ingredients:

- 1 lb chicken tenders
- 1 cup almond flour
- 1/2 cup grated parmesan cheese
- 1 large egg
- 1 tbsp olive oil
- 1 tsp garlic powder
- 1 tsp paprika
- 1/2 tsp salt
- 1/2 tsp black pepper

Instructions:

1. Set your oven to 400°F (200°C) and cover a baking sheet with parchment paper.
2. In a shallow bowl, mix together the almond flour, parmesan cheese, garlic powder, paprika, salt, and black pepper.
3. In another shallow bowl, beat the egg.
4. Dip each chicken tender into the beaten egg, then coat it with the almond flour mixture, pressing it to adhere.
5. Place the coated chicken tenders on the prepared baking sheet.
6. Drizzle with olive oil and bake for 20-25 minutes or until golden brown and cooked through.
7. Serve with your favorite dipping sauce.

Almond Flour Veggie Patties

Ingredients:

- 2 cups grated zucchini
- 1 cup grated carrots
- 1 cup almond flour
- 1/4 cup grated parmesan cheese
- 2 large eggs
- 2 tbsp chopped fresh parsley
- 1 tsp garlic powder
- 1/2 tsp salt
- 1/2 tsp black pepper
- 2 tbsp olive oil for frying

Instructions:

1. In a sizable bowl, mix the grated zucchini, grated carrots, almond flour, parmesan cheese, eggs, parsley, garlic powder, salt, and black pepper together.
2. Form the mixture into 8 patties.
3. Heat the olive oil in a large skillet over medium heat.
4. Cook the veggie patties for 3-4 minutes on each side, or until golden brown and crispy.
5. Serve warm with a side salad or in a sandwich.

Almond Flour Flatbreads

Ingredients:

- 2 cups almond flour
- 2 large eggs
- 1/4 cup water
- 1 tbsp olive oil
- 1/2 tsp salt

Instructions:

1. In a sizable bowl, combine the almond flour, eggs, water, olive oil, and salt until the dough takes shape.
2. Divide the dough into 6 equal portions and roll each portion into a ball.
3. Place each ball between two sheets of parchment paper and roll it into a thin circle.
4. Heat a non-stick skillet over medium heat and cook each flatbread for 1-2 minutes on each side, or until lightly browned and cooked through.
5. Serve warm with your favorite fillings or as a side to your meal.

Almond Flour Pasta

Ingredients:

- 2 cups almond flour
- 1/4 cup tapioca flour
- 1/4 cup psyllium husk powder
- 1/2 tsp salt
- 3 large eggs
- 1 tbsp olive oil

Instructions:

1. In a sizable bowl, mix the almond flour, tapioca flour, psyllium husk powder, and salt together.
2. Make a well in the center and add the eggs and olive oil.
3. Mix until a dough forms, then knead for a few minutes until smooth.
4. Divide the dough into 4 equal portions and roll each portion into a thin sheet.
5. Cut the sheets into your desired pasta shape (e.g., fettuccine, spaghetti).
6. Bring a large pot of salted water to a boil and cook the pasta for 2-3 minutes or until al dente.
7. Serve with your favorite sauce.

Almond Flour Soup Thickener

Ingredients:

- 2-3 tablespoons almond flour
- 1 cup cold water or broth
- Your favorite soup recipe

Instructions:

1. In a small bowl, whisk together the almond flour and cold water or broth until smooth.
2. Add the mixture to your soup and stir well.
3. Bring the soup to a boil and then reduce heat to a simmer.
4. Let the soup cook for an additional 5-10 minutes, stirring occasionally, until thickened to your desired consistency.
5. Serve hot and enjoy your thick and creamy soup!
6. You can also use almond flour as a substitute for other thickeners such as cornstarch or wheat flour in various recipes like stews, gravies, and sauces.

Dinner Recipes Using Almond Flour

Almond-Crusted Salmon

Ingredients:

- 4 salmon fillets
- 1 cup almond flour
- 1/4 cup grated Parmesan cheese
- 1 tbsp fresh parsley, chopped
- 1 tsp garlic powder
- 1 tsp lemon zest
- Salt and pepper to taste
- 2 tbsp olive oil

Instructions:

1. Set your oven to 400°F (200°C) and cover a baking sheet with parchment paper.
2. In a bowl, mix together the almond flour, Parmesan cheese, parsley, garlic powder, lemon zest, salt, and pepper.
3. Brush each salmon fillet with olive oil.
4. Press the almond flour mixture onto the top of each fillet to coat.
5. Place the fillets on the prepared baking sheet and bake for 12-15 minutes, or until the salmon is cooked through and the crust is golden brown.
6. Serve with a side of vegetables or a fresh salad.

Almond Flour Meatballs

Ingredients:

- 1 lb ground beef or turkey
- 1/2 cup almond flour
- 1/4 cup grated Parmesan cheese
- 1 large egg
- 1 tbsp fresh parsley, chopped
- 1 tsp garlic powder
- 1 tsp onion powder
- Salt and pepper to taste
- 2 tbsp olive oil

Instructions:

1. Heat your oven to 375°F (190°C) and place parchment paper on a baking sheet.
2. Mix the ground meat, almond flour, Parmesan cheese, egg, parsley, garlic powder, onion powder, salt, and pepper together in a large bowl.
3. Form the mixture into 12-16 meatballs.
4. Heat the olive oil in a large skillet over medium heat and brown the meatballs on all sides, about 5-7 minutes.

5. Transfer the meatballs to the prepared baking sheet and bake for an additional 10-15 minutes, or until cooked through.
6. Serve with marinara sauce and spaghetti squash or zucchini noodles.

Almond Flour Lasagna

Ingredients:

- 1 lb ground beef or turkey
- 1 cup marinara sauce
- 2 cups ricotta cheese
- 2 cups shredded mozzarella cheese
- 1/2 cup grated Parmesan cheese
- 2 large eggs
- 1 cup almond flour
- 1/4 cup coconut flour
- 1 tsp garlic powder
- 1 tsp onion powder
- Salt and pepper to taste

Instructions:

1. Warm your oven to 375°F (190°C) and lightly grease a 9x13-inch baking dish.
2. In a skillet, cook the ground meat over medium heat until browned. Drain excess fat and stir in marinara sauce.
3. In a bowl, mix together the ricotta cheese, 1 cup of mozzarella cheese, Parmesan cheese, eggs, almond flour, coconut flour, garlic powder, onion powder, salt, and pepper.
4. Spread a thin layer of the meat sauce on the bottom of the baking dish.

5. Layer with the ricotta mixture, followed by more meat sauce. Repeat layers, ending with meat sauce.
6. Top with the remaining 1 cup of mozzarella cheese.
7. Cover with foil and bake for 25 minutes, then remove the foil and bake for an additional 10-15 minutes, or until the cheese is golden and bubbly.
8. Allow to cool for 10 minutes before serving.

Almond Flour Battered Fish

Ingredients:

- 4 white fish fillets (such as cod or tilapia)
- 1 cup almond flour
- 1/4 cup tapioca flour
- 1 tsp baking powder
- 1 tsp garlic powder
- 1/2 tsp paprika
- Salt and pepper to taste
- 2 large eggs
- 1/4 cup water
- Vegetable oil for frying

Instructions:

1. In a shallow bowl, mix together the almond flour, tapioca flour, baking powder, garlic powder, paprika, salt, and pepper.
2. In another bowl, whisk together the eggs and water.
3. Heat vegetable oil in a large skillet over medium-high heat.
4. Dip each fish fillet in the egg mixture, then coat it with the almond flour mixture.
5. Fry the fish in the hot oil for 3-4 minutes on each side, or until golden brown and cooked through.
6. Drain on paper towels and serve with lemon wedges and tartar sauce.

Almond Flour Stuffed Peppers

Ingredients:

- 4 bell peppers, tops cut off and seeds removed
- 1 lb ground beef or turkey
- 1/2 cup almond flour
- 1/2 cup cooked quinoa
- 1 cup marinara sauce
- 1/2 cup shredded mozzarella cheese
- 1/4 cup grated Parmesan cheese
- 1 tsp garlic powder
- 1 tsp onion powder
- Salt and pepper to taste
- 1 tbsp olive oil

Instructions:

1. Heat your oven to 375°F (190°C) and lightly coat a baking dish with grease.
2. In a skillet, cook the ground meat over medium heat until browned. Drain excess fat.
3. Mix the cooked meat, almond flour, cooked quinoa, marinara sauce, mozzarella, Parmesan, garlic powder, onion powder, salt, and pepper together in a large bowl.
4. Stuff each bell pepper with the meat mixture and place them in the prepared baking dish.

5. Drizzle with olive oil and cover with foil.
6. Bake for 30 minutes, then remove the foil and bake for an additional 10-15 minutes, or until the peppers are tender and the filling is heated through.
7. Serve hot.

Almond Flour Chicken Parmesan

Ingredients:

- 4 boneless, skinless chicken breasts
- 1 cup almond flour
- 1/2 cup grated Parmesan cheese
- 1 tsp garlic powder
- 1 tsp Italian seasoning
- Salt and pepper to taste
- 2 large eggs
- 1 cup marinara sauce
- 1 cup shredded mozzarella cheese
- 2 tbsp olive oil

Instructions:

1. Set your oven to 400°F (200°C) and apply grease to a baking dish.
2. In a shallow bowl, mix together the almond flour, Parmesan cheese, garlic powder, Italian seasoning, salt, and pepper.
3. In another bowl, beat the eggs.
4. Dip each chicken breast in the eggs, then coat with the almond flour mixture.
5. Heat olive oil in a large skillet over medium heat and brown the chicken on both sides, about 3-4 minutes per side.

6. Place the browned chicken in the prepared baking dish, and top with marinara sauce and mozzarella cheese.
7. Bake for 20-25 minutes, or until the chicken is cooked through and the cheese is melted and bubbly.
8. Serve with gluten-free pasta or a side salad.

Almond Flour Zucchini Fries

Ingredients:

- 4 medium zucchinis, cut into fries
- 1 cup almond flour
- 1/4 cup grated Parmesan cheese
- 1 tsp garlic powder
- 1 tsp paprika
- 1/2 tsp salt
- 1/2 tsp black pepper
- 2 large eggs
- Olive oil spray

Instructions:

1. Adjust your oven to 425°F (220°C) and place parchment paper on a baking sheet.
2. In a shallow bowl, mix together the almond flour, Parmesan cheese, garlic powder, paprika, salt, and black pepper.
3. In another bowl, beat the eggs.
4. Dip each zucchini fry in the eggs, then coat with the almond flour mixture.
5. Arrange the zucchini fries on the prepared baking sheet and spray with olive oil.
6. Bake for 20-25 minutes or until golden brown and crispy, turning halfway through.
7. Serve with your favorite dipping sauce.

Almond Flour Meatloaf

Ingredients:

- 1 lb ground beef or turkey
- 1/2 cup almond flour
- 1/4 cup grated Parmesan cheese
- 1 large egg
- 1/4 cup milk or almond milk
- 1 tbsp Worcestershire sauce
- 1 tsp garlic powder
- 1 tsp onion powder
- Salt and pepper to taste
- 1/2 cup ketchup

Instructions:

1. Warm your oven to 375°F (190°C) and lightly grease a loaf pan.
2. Mix the ground meat, almond flour, Parmesan cheese, egg, milk, Worcestershire sauce, garlic powder, onion powder, salt, and pepper together in a large bowl.
3. Press the mixture into the prepared loaf pan and spread the ketchup evenly over the top.
4. Bake for 45-55 minutes, or until the meatloaf is cooked through and the internal temperature reaches 160°F (70°C).
5. Let the meatloaf rest for 10 minutes before slicing and serving.

Almond Flour Cauliflower Pizza

Ingredients:

- 1 medium head of cauliflower, riced
- 1 cup almond flour
- 1/2 cup grated Parmesan cheese
- 2 large eggs
- 1 tsp garlic powder
- 1 tsp Italian seasoning
- Salt and pepper to taste
- Your favorite pizza toppings

Instructions:

1. Heat your oven to 425°F (220°C) and cover a baking sheet with parchment paper.
2. Steam the riced cauliflower for 5 minutes, then drain and squeeze out as much water as possible using a clean kitchen towel.
3. Mix the cauliflower, almond flour, Parmesan cheese, eggs, garlic powder, Italian seasoning, salt, and pepper together in a large bowl.
4. Press the mixture into a thin, even circle on the prepared baking sheet.
5. Bake for 15-20 minutes, or until the crust is golden brown and firm.

6. Remove from the oven, add your favorite pizza toppings, and return to the oven for an additional 10-15 minutes, or until the toppings are cooked to your liking.
7. Slice and serve.

Almond Flour Gnocchi

Ingredients:

- 1 cup almond flour
- 1 cup ricotta cheese
- 1/2 cup grated Parmesan cheese
- 1 large egg
- 1/4 cup tapioca flour
- 1/2 tsp salt
- Your favorite pasta sauce

Instructions:

1. Combine the almond flour, ricotta cheese, Parmesan cheese, egg, tapioca flour, and salt in a large bowl and mix until a dough forms.
2. Divide the dough into four equal portions and roll each portion into a long rope about 1/2 inch in diameter.
3. Cut the ropes into 1-inch pieces to form the gnocchi.
4. Bring a large pot of salted water to a boil and cook the gnocchi in batches for 2-3 minutes, or until they float to the surface.
5. Remove with a slotted spoon and transfer to a plate.
6. Serve the gnocchi with your favorite pasta sauce and a sprinkle of Parmesan cheese.
7. Dessert Recipes Using Almond Flour

Almond Flour Chocolate Chip Cookies

Ingredients:

- 2 cups almond flour
- 1/2 cup coconut oil, melted
- 1/2 cup brown sugar
- 1/4 cup granulated sugar
- 1 large egg
- 1 tsp vanilla extract
- 1/2 tsp baking soda
- 1/4 tsp salt
- 1 cup chocolate chips

Instructions:

1. Set your oven to 350°F (175°C) and place parchment paper on a baking sheet.
2. Combine the almond flour, coconut oil, brown sugar, granulated sugar, egg, and vanilla extract in a large bowl and mix thoroughly until well blended.
3. Add the baking soda and salt, and mix until incorporated.
4. Fold in the chocolate chips.
5. Scoop tablespoon-sized balls of dough onto the prepared baking sheet, spacing them about 2 inches apart.

6. Bake for 10-12 minutes, or until the edges are golden brown.
7. Allow the cookies to cool on the baking sheet for 5 minutes before transferring them to a wire rack to cool completely.

Almond Flour Brownies

Ingredients:

- 1 cup almond flour
- 1/2 cup cocoa powder
- 1/2 cup melted coconut oil
- 1/2 cup brown sugar
- 1/4 cup granulated sugar
- 2 large eggs
- 1 tsp vanilla extract
- 1/4 tsp salt
- 1/2 tsp baking powder

Instructions:

1. Warm your oven to 350°F (175°C) and lightly coat an 8x8-inch baking dish with grease.
2. In a big bowl, blend almond flour, cocoa powder, melted coconut oil, brown sugar, granulated sugar, eggs, vanilla extract, salt, and baking powder until the mixture is well combined.
3. Pour the batter into the prepared baking dish and spread it evenly.
4. Bake for 20-25 minutes, or until a toothpick inserted into the center comes out clean.
5. Allow the brownies to cool in the baking dish before cutting them into squares.

Almond Flour Cupcakes

Ingredients:

- 2 cups almond flour
- 1/4 cup coconut flour
- 1/2 cup coconut oil, melted
- 1/2 cup honey or maple syrup
- 4 large eggs
- 1 tsp vanilla extract
- 1/2 tsp baking soda
- 1/4 tsp salt

Instructions:

1. Set your oven to 350°F (175°C) and place cupcake liners in a muffin tin.
2. In a big bowl, combine almond flour, coconut flour, melted coconut oil, honey or maple syrup, eggs, vanilla extract, baking soda, and salt until thoroughly mixed.
3. Divide the batter evenly among the cupcake liners.
4. Bake for 18-22 minutes, or until a toothpick inserted into the center comes out clean.
5. Allow the cupcakes to cool in the tin for 5 minutes before transferring them to a wire rack to cool completely.

Almond Flour Cheesecake Crust

Ingredients:

- 1 1/2 cups almond flour
- 1/4 cup melted butter
- 2 tbsp granulated sugar
- 1/2 tsp vanilla extract

Instructions:

1. Heat your oven to 350°F (175°C) and lightly grease a 9-inch springform pan.
2. In a medium bowl, mix together the almond flour, melted butter, granulated sugar, and vanilla extract until well combined.
3. Press the mixture evenly into the bottom of the prepared pan.
4. Bake for 8-10 minutes, or until the crust is lightly golden.
5. Allow the crust to cool before adding your cheesecake filling.

Almond Flour Banana Bread

Ingredients:

- 2 cups almond flour
- 1/4 cup coconut flour
- 3 ripe bananas, mashed
- 1/4 cup melted coconut oil
- 1/4 cup honey or maple syrup
- 3 large eggs
- 1 tsp vanilla extract
- 1/2 tsp baking soda
- 1/4 tsp salt

Instructions:

1. Warm your oven to 350°F (175°C) and coat a loaf pan with grease.
2. In a big bowl, blend almond flour, coconut flour, mashed bananas, melted coconut oil, honey or maple syrup, eggs, vanilla extract, baking soda, and salt until the mixture is well combined.
3. Pour the batter into the prepared loaf pan and spread it evenly.
4. Bake for 45-55 minutes, or until a toothpick inserted into the center comes out clean.
5. Allow the banana bread to cool in the pan for 10 minutes before transferring it to a wire rack to cool completely.

Almond Flour Macaroons

Ingredients:

- 2 cups shredded coconut
- 1 cup almond flour
- 1/2 cup sweetened condensed milk
- 1 tsp vanilla extract
- 1/4 tsp salt

Instructions:

1. Heat your oven to 350°F (175°C) and cover a baking sheet with parchment paper.
2. In a big bowl, combine shredded coconut, almond flour, sweetened condensed milk, vanilla extract, and salt until everything is well blended.
3. Scoop tablespoon-sized balls of the mixture onto the prepared baking sheet, spacing them about 2 inches apart.
4. Bake for 12-15 minutes, or until the macaroons are golden brown.
5. Allow the macaroons to cool on the baking sheet for 5 minutes before transferring them to a wire rack to cool completely.

Almond Flour Donuts

Ingredients:

- 2 cups almond flour
- 1/4 cup coconut flour
- 1/2 cup coconut oil, melted
- 1/2 cup honey or maple syrup
- 4 large eggs
- 1 tsp vanilla extract
- 1/2 tsp baking soda
- 1/4 tsp salt
- 1/2 tsp ground cinnamon

Instructions:

1. Heat your oven to 350°F (175°C) and lightly coat a donut pan with grease.
2. In a big bowl, blend almond flour, coconut flour, melted coconut oil, honey or maple syrup, eggs, vanilla extract, baking soda, salt, and ground cinnamon until thoroughly mixed.
3. Spoon the batter into the prepared donut pan, filling each cavity about 2/3 full.
4. Bake for 15-18 minutes, or until a toothpick inserted into the center comes out clean.
5. Allow the donuts to cool in the pan for 5 minutes before transferring them to a wire rack to cool completely.

Almond Flour Scones

Ingredients:

- 2 cups almond flour
- 1/4 cup coconut flour
- 1/4 cup cold butter, cubed
- 1/4 cup honey or maple syrup
- 2 large eggs
- 1 tsp vanilla extract
- 1/2 tsp baking soda
- 1/4 tsp salt
- 1/2 cup dried fruit or chocolate chips (optional)

Instructions:

1. Warm your oven to 350°F (175°C) and cover a baking sheet with parchment paper.
2. In a big bowl, combine almond flour, coconut flour, cold butter, honey or maple syrup, eggs, vanilla extract, baking soda, and salt until a dough is formed.
3. Fold in the dried fruit or chocolate chips, if using.
4. Turn the dough onto the prepared baking sheet and shape it into a round disc about 1 inch thick.
5. Cut the disc into 8 wedges and separate them slightly.

6. Bake for 18-22 minutes, or until the scones are golden brown.
7. Allow the scones to cool on the baking sheet for 5 minutes before transferring them to a wire rack to cool completely.

Snack Recipes Using Almond Flour

Almond Flour Crackers

Ingredients:

- 2 cups almond flour
- 2 tbsp ground flaxseed
- 1/4 tsp sea salt
- 1 large egg
- 2 tbsp olive oil
- 1 tsp dried herbs (optional)

Instructions:

1. Set your oven to 350°F (175°C) and place parchment paper on a baking sheet.
2. Combine the almond flour, ground flaxseed, and sea salt in a large bowl.
3. Add the egg and olive oil, and mix until a dough forms.
4. Roll the dough between two sheets of parchment paper to 1/8-inch thickness.
5. Remove the top sheet of parchment paper and cut the dough into squares.

6. Transfer the parchment paper with the cut dough onto the baking sheet.
7. Bake for 12-15 minutes, or until the edges are golden brown.
8. Allow the crackers to cool completely before breaking them apart and serving.

Almond Flour Energy Balls

Ingredients:

- 1 cup almond flour
- 1/2 cup rolled oats
- 1/4 cup almond butter
- 1/4 cup honey or maple syrup
- 1/4 cup chocolate chips
- 1 tsp vanilla extract
- 1/4 tsp sea salt

Instructions:

1. Mix the almond flour, rolled oats, almond butter, honey or maple syrup, chocolate chips, vanilla extract, and sea salt together in a large bowl.
2. Mix until well combined and a dough forms.
3. Roll the mixture into tablespoon-sized balls and place them on a baking sheet lined with parchment paper.
4. Refrigerate for at least 30 minutes before serving.

Almond Flour Pretzels

Ingredients:

- 2 cups almond flour
- 1/4 cup coconut flour
- 1/4 cup psyllium husk powder
- 1 tsp baking powder
- 1/2 tsp sea salt
- 1 cup boiling water
- 1 large egg, beaten (for egg wash)
- Coarse salt (for topping)

Instructions:

1. Heat your oven to 375°F (190°C) and cover a baking sheet with parchment paper.
2. Combine the almond flour, coconut flour, psyllium husk powder, baking powder, and sea salt in a large bowl and mix thoroughly.
3. Add the boiling water and mix until a dough forms.
4. Divide the dough into 8 equal portions and roll each portion into a long rope.
5. Shape each rope into a pretzel and place them on the prepared baking sheet.
6. Brush the beaten egg over the pretzels and sprinkle with coarse salt.
7. Bake for 20-25 minutes, or until golden brown.
8. Allow the pretzels to cool slightly before serving.

Almond Flour Granola Bars

Ingredients:

- 2 cups rolled oats
- 1 cup almond flour
- 1/2 cup honey or maple syrup
- 1/2 cup almond butter
- 1/4 cup coconut oil, melted
- 1/4 cup chopped nuts
- 1/4 cup dried fruit
- 1 tsp vanilla extract
- 1/4 tsp sea salt

Instructions:

1. Set your oven to 350°F (175°C) and place parchment paper in an 8x8-inch baking dish.
2. Mix the rolled oats, almond flour, honey or maple syrup, almond butter, melted coconut oil, chopped nuts, dried fruit, vanilla extract, and sea salt together in a large bowl.
3. Mix until well combined and press the mixture evenly into the prepared baking dish.
4. Bake for 20-25 minutes, or until golden brown.
5. Allow the granola bars to cool completely in the baking dish before cutting them into squares.

Almond Flour Cheese Straws

Ingredients:

- 2 cups almond flour
- 1 cup grated cheddar cheese
- 1/4 cup grated Parmesan cheese
- 1/4 cup cold butter, cubed
- 1 large egg
- 1/2 tsp garlic powder
- 1/2 tsp paprika
- 1/4 tsp sea salt

Instructions:

1. Warm your oven to 350°F (190°C) and cover a baking sheet with parchment paper.
2. In a food processor, combine the almond flour, grated cheddar cheese, grated Parmesan cheese, cold butter, garlic powder, paprika, and sea salt.
3. Pulse until the mixture resembles coarse crumbs.
4. Add the egg and pulse until a dough forms.
5. Roll the dough between two sheets of parchment paper to 1/4-inch thickness.
6. Cut the dough into strips and place them on the prepared baking sheet.
7. Bake for 12-15 minutes, or until golden brown.
8. Allow the cheese straws to cool completely before serving.

Almond Flour Protein Bites

Ingredients:

- 1 cup almond flour
- 1/2 cup protein powder
- 1/4 cup almond butter
- 1/4 cup honey or maple syrup
- 1/4 cup chocolate chips
- 1 tsp vanilla extract
- 1/4 tsp sea salt

Instructions:

1. Mix the almond flour, protein powder, almond butter, honey or maple syrup, chocolate chips, vanilla extract, and sea salt together in a large bowl.
2. Mix until well combined and a dough forms.
3. Roll the mixture into tablespoon-sized balls and place them on a baking sheet lined with parchment paper.
4. Refrigerate for at least 30 minutes before serving.

Almond Flour Popcorn Chicken

Ingredients:

- 1 lb chicken breast, cut into bite-sized pieces
- 1 cup almond flour
- 1/2 cup grated Parmesan cheese
- 1 tsp garlic powder
- 1 tsp paprika
- 1/2 tsp sea salt
- 1/2 tsp black pepper
- 2 large eggs, beaten
- Oil for frying

Instructions:

1. Mix the almond flour, grated Parmesan cheese, garlic powder, paprika, sea salt, and black pepper together in a large bowl.
2. Dip each piece of chicken into the beaten eggs, then coat with the almond flour mixture.
3. Heat oil in a large skillet over medium-high heat.
4. Fry the chicken in batches until golden brown and cooked through, about 4-5 minutes per side.
5. Remove with a slotted spoon and drain on paper towels.
6. Serve immediately with your favorite dipping sauce.

Almond Flour Onion Rings

Ingredients:

- 2 large onions, sliced into rings
- 1 cup almond flour
- 1/2 cup grated Parmesan cheese
- 1 tsp garlic powder
- 1 tsp paprika
- 1/2 tsp sea salt
- 2 large eggs, beaten
- Oil for frying

Instructions:

1. Mix the almond flour, grated Parmesan cheese, garlic powder, paprika, and sea salt together in a large bowl.
2. Dip each onion ring into the beaten eggs, then coat with the almond flour mixture.
3. Heat oil in a large skillet over medium-high heat.
4. Fry the onion rings in batches until golden brown and crispy, about 2-3 minutes per side.
5. Remove with a slotted spoon and drain on paper towels.
6. Serve immediately with your favorite dipping sauce.

Almond Flour Crisps

Ingredients:

- 2 cups almond flour
- 1/4 cup olive oil
- 1 large egg
- 1/2 tsp sea salt
- 1/2 tsp garlic powder
- 1/2 tsp paprika

Instructions:

1. Warm your oven to 350°F (175°C) and cover a baking sheet with parchment paper.
2. In a big bowl, mix together almond flour, olive oil, egg, sea salt, garlic powder, and paprika.
3. Mix until a dough forms.
4. Roll the dough between two sheets of parchment paper to 1/8-inch thickness.
5. Remove the top sheet of parchment paper and cut the dough into small squares or circles.
6. Transfer the parchment paper with the cut dough onto the baking sheet.
7. Bake for 10-12 minutes, or until the crisps are golden brown.
8. Allow the crisps to cool completely before serving.

Almond Flour Fruit Tarts

Ingredients:

For the Crust:

- 1 1/2 cups almond flour
- 1/4 cup melted butter
- 2 tbsp granulated sugar
- 1/2 tsp vanilla extract

For the Filling:

- 1 cup Greek yogurt or coconut yogurt
- 2 tbsp honey or maple syrup
- 1 tsp vanilla extract

For the Topping:

- Fresh fruit (such as berries, kiwi, or mango), sliced

Instructions:

1. Set your oven to 350°F (175°C) and lightly grease a muffin tin or tartlet pan.
2. In a medium bowl, mix together the almond flour, melted butter, granulated sugar, and vanilla extract until well combined.
3. Press the mixture evenly into the bottom and up the sides of the prepared muffin tin or tartlet pan to form crusts.

4. Bake for 8-10 minutes, or until the crusts are lightly golden. Allow to cool completely.
5. In another bowl, mix together the Greek yogurt or coconut yogurt, honey or maple syrup, and vanilla extract until smooth.
6. Spoon the yogurt mixture into the cooled crusts.
7. Top with sliced fresh fruit.
8. Serve immediately or refrigerate until ready to serve.

6 Step-by-Step Plan to Start Incorporating Almond Flour into Your Recipes

Incorporating almond flour into your recipes is a great way to add a nutty and delicious flavor while also boosting the nutritional value of your dishes. Here is a step-by-step plan to help you get started with using almond flour in your cooking and baking:

Step 1: Choose the Right Almond Flour

When you're just getting started with almond flour, it's essential to pick the right type to suit your needs and preferences.

1. **Start with Blanched Almond Flour**

    As a beginner, you'll find blanched almond flour to be the most versatile option. This flour is made from almonds that have had their skins removed through a blanching process. The result is a finer, lighter flour that blends seamlessly into most recipes, providing a smoother consistency. This makes it ideal for baked goods like cakes, cookies, and bread where you want a delicate texture.

2. **Consider Unblanched Almond Flour**

   If you're open to experimenting with textures, consider trying unblanched almond flour. This type includes the almond skins, giving the flour a slightly coarser texture and a speckled appearance. It can add a rustic, hearty feel to your baked goods and is excellent for recipes where a bit of texture is welcome, such as in certain cookies or crusts.

3. **Check Freshness**

   Freshness is key to achieving the best results with almond flour. Always inspect the flour for a light, even color and a pleasant nutty aroma. Avoid any almond flour that has a yellowish hue or smells off, as these are signs of rancidity. Fresh almond flour ensures your recipes taste their best and maintain optimal nutritional value.

4. **Organic and Non-GMO Options**

   Whenever possible, choose organic and non-GMO almond flour. Organic flour is made without synthetic pesticides or fertilizers, making it healthier for you and the environment. Non-GMO flour ensures the almonds are not genetically modified, offering a more natural product. While these options may cost a bit more, they provide better quality and peace of mind about what you're consuming.

By carefully selecting the right almond flour, you set a solid foundation for creating delicious and nutritious recipes that will delight your taste buds and support your health goals.

Step 2: Understand its Properties

Understanding the unique properties of almond flour is crucial for achieving the best results in your cooking and baking endeavors.

1. **Denser and Moister**

   Almond flour is naturally denser and moister than traditional wheat flour because it is made from ground almonds, which contain more oil and less starch. This density and moisture can result in baked goods that are heavier and more moist.

   For instance, cakes and muffins may have a richer texture and might not have the same light, airy quality you're used to with wheat flour. You may need to adjust your expectations and possibly tweak your recipes slightly, such as reducing the amount of oil or adding an extra egg to balance the moisture.

2. **Lack of Gluten**

   One of the most significant differences between almond flour and wheat flour is the lack of gluten. Gluten is the protein in wheat that gives dough its elasticity and helps it rise. Without gluten, your baked goods may not rise as much and will have a denser texture.

   To counter this, you might need to use additional binding agents, such as eggs or xanthan gum, to help provide structure. You can also combine almond flour with other gluten-free flour, like coconut flour or tapioca starch, to achieve a better texture.

3. **Storage Tips**

   Proper storage of almond flour is crucial for maintaining freshness and extending shelf life. Keep it in an airtight container to protect it from moisture and air, which can lead to spoilage. Storing almond flour in the refrigerator or freezer is ideal, as the cold slows down the oxidation of the natural oils in the almonds. When you're ready to use it, allow the almond flour to reach room temperature to prevent clumping. This ensures that it blends smoothly into your recipes for consistent results.

By understanding and adapting to the properties of almond flour, you can make delicious, nutritious dishes that take full advantage of its unique characteristics.

Step 3: Start with Simple Recipes

If you're new to using almond flour, it's a great idea to start with simple recipes that only require a small amount of flour. This approach allows you to familiarize yourself with how almond flour behaves in various baking applications and helps you understand any adjustments you might need to make for optimal results.

Some easy and delicious recipes to try include:

- *Almond Flour Pancakes*: These pancakes are an excellent option for breakfast or brunch. They are light, fluffy, and gluten-free, making them a perfect choice for those with dietary restrictions. Plus, you can customize them by adding fruits like blueberries or bananas, or even a sprinkle of cinnamon for extra flavor.
- *Almond Flour Chocolate Chip Cookies*: If you're looking to satisfy your sweet tooth, these cookies are a must-try! Made with almond flour and dark chocolate chips, they offer a rich flavor and chewy texture. You can also experiment by adding nuts or dried fruit for an added crunch and taste.

- *Almond Flour Banana Bread*: This classic treat gets a healthy twist with the addition of almond flour. The result is a moist and flavorful loaf that's perfect for breakfast or as a snack. You can enhance the recipe by adding walnuts, chocolate chips, or even a swirl of peanut butter for more richness.

As you gain more experience with almond flour, feel free to experiment by using it in more complex recipes. You might consider substituting it for wheat flour in your favorite traditional dishes, such as bread, muffins, or even pizza crust. Just remember that almond flour has different absorption properties and may require adjustments in the liquid content of your recipes. Happy baking!

Step 4: Substitute Almond Flour in Traditional Recipes

Venturing into the world of almond flour substitutions can be a game-changer for your kitchen creations. Almond flour is not only a gluten-free alternative but also adds a rich, nutty flavor and a boost of nutrition to your dishes. Here's how you can start substituting almond flour in traditional recipes with ease and confidence.

1. **Partial Substitution**

   Starting Small:

When you're new to using almond flour, it's best to start with partial substitution. Replace up to 25% of the wheat flour in your recipes with almond flour. This method allows you to enjoy the health benefits of almond flour without drastically altering the texture and structure of your baked goods.

Example:

For a recipe that calls for 2 cups of all-purpose flour, substitute 1/2 cup of it with almond flour. This way, you retain the familiarity of your favorite recipes while subtly enhancing them with the goodness of almonds.

2. Adjusting Leavening Agents

Balancing Act:

Almond flour is denser than wheat flour, which means it doesn't rise as much on its own. When using more almond flour or going entirely gluten-free with it, you might need to tweak the leavening agents to achieve the desired rise and fluffiness in your baked goods.

Tips:

1. *Extra Egg*: Adding an extra egg can help provide structure and moisture.
2. *Additional Baking Powder*: Increase the baking powder by about 1/4 to 1/2 teaspoon per cup of almond flour.

3. *Binder Ingredients*: Ingredients like xanthan gum or psyllium husk can also be added to mimic the elasticity of gluten.

Example:

For a cake recipe that uses 1 cup of wheat flour and 1 teaspoon of baking powder, if you switch to 100% almond flour, you might use 1 1/4 cups almond flour and 1 1/2 teaspoons of baking powder, plus an extra egg for better structure.

3. **Savory Applications**

   Crunchy Coatings:

Almond flour isn't just for sweet treats; it shines in savory dishes too. Use it as a breading for meats and vegetables. It creates a beautifully crispy and flavorful coating that's both nutritious and satisfying.

Instructions:

1. *For Breading Meats*: Dip your chicken, fish, or pork chops in beaten egg, then coat them in almond flour mixed with your favorite seasonings. Pan-fry or bake until golden brown.
2. *For Vegetables*: Toss sliced veggies like zucchini or eggplant in almond flour and bake or fry as desired.

Thickening Soups and Sauces:

Almond flour can also be a fantastic thickener for soups and sauces, adding a subtle nutty flavor.

Instructions:

1. ***For Soups***: Stir in a few tablespoons of almond flour toward the end of cooking to thicken the broth.
2. ***For Sauces***: Whisk almond flour into your sauce base, cooking until it reaches the desired consistency.

By incorporating almond flour into your traditional recipes, you not only make them healthier but also add a deliciously nutty twist that's sure to impress. Start experimenting today and take delight in the versatile and nutritious world of almond flour.

Step 5: Appreciate the Benefits

In addition to its versatility in cooking and baking, almond flour also offers a wide range of health benefits. Here are some key reasons why you should consider incorporating almond flour into your diet:

- *Gluten-free*: Almond flour is naturally gluten-free, making it a great option for those with celiac disease or gluten sensitivity.

- *Low glycemic index*: Compared to other flours, almond flour has a lower glycemic index, meaning it won't cause a spike in blood sugar levels after consumption.
- *Good for heart health*: Almond flour is high in healthy fats, including monounsaturated and polyunsaturated fats. These types of fats have been linked to reducing the risk of heart disease.
- *Helps with weight management*: Due to its high protein and fiber content, using almond flour in your recipes can help you feel full for longer periods, potentially aiding in weight management.
- *Rich in nutrients*: Almond flour is rich in various vitamins and minerals such as vitamin E, magnesium, and manganese. These nutrients are essential for maintaining overall health and well-being.

Incorporating almond flour into your diet not only adds nutritional value but also makes meals more flavorful and satisfying. So go ahead and experiment with new recipes or simply substitute regular flour with almond flour in your favorite dishes. Enjoy the delicious and nutritious world of almond flour.

Step 6: Experiment and Innovate

The adventure of cooking with almond flour is just beginning! Embrace the opportunity to experiment and innovate in your kitchen. Almond flour offers endless possibilities for both sweet and savory dishes, and there's a whole community of fellow enthusiasts ready to support and inspire you. Here's how you can dive deep into the world of almond flour, experiment boldly, and document your journey for continuous improvement.

1. **Try New Recipes**

   Step Out of Your Comfort Zone:

   Don't hesitate to try new and exciting recipes with almond flour. It's a versatile ingredient that works wonderfully in both sweet and savory dishes. Here are some suggestions to get you started:

   Sweet Delights:

   - *Almond Flour Bread*: A gluten-free option that's perfect for sandwiches or toast.
   - *Almond Flour Cakes*: Moist and flavorful, with a subtle nutty taste that pairs well with fruits and spices.
   - *Almond Flour Brownies*: Rich, fudgy, and packed with a delightful almond flavor.

2. **Savory Treats:**
   - *Quiche Crusts*: Use almond flour for a gluten-free, nutty crust that complements a variety of fillings.

- *Savory Muffins*: Combine almond flour with cheese, herbs, and veggies for a nutritious snack or breakfast.
- *Almond Flour Pizza Crust*: A healthy alternative to traditional pizza dough that's both crispy and delicious.

3. **Join Communities**

Connect and Share:

The journey is always more enjoyable with companions. Look for online groups or forums where people share their almond flour recipes and tips. Engaging with these communities offers numerous benefits:

- *Inspiration*: Discover new and creative ways to use almond flour.
- *Support*: Get advice and encouragement from fellow almond flour enthusiasts.
- *Sharing*: Exchange your own experiences and recipes, helping others while learning from them.

Where to Look:

- *Social Media*: Platforms like Instagram, Facebook, and Pinterest are brimming with food bloggers and home cooks sharing their almond flour creations.

- *Blogs*: Follow baking and cooking blogs that specialize in gluten-free or almond flour recipes for regular updates and tips.
- *Forums*: Join forums like Reddit's gluten-free or keto subreddits to find a supportive community.

4. Keep a Cooking Journal

Document Your Journey:

Keeping a cooking journal is a fantastic way to track your progress and refine your almond flour techniques. Here's how to make the most of it:

What to Note Down:

- *Recipes Tried*: List the recipes you've attempted, along with any specific changes you made.
- *Successes and Failures*: Document what worked well and what didn't. This helps you avoid repeating mistakes and builds your confidence.
- *Adjustments*: Note any ingredient substitutions or proportion changes you made and their effects on the final product.
- *Tasting Notes*: Record the taste, texture, and overall satisfaction of the dish. This helps you

remember what you enjoyed and what could use improvement.

5. **Benefits of a Cooking Journal:**
   - *Refinement*: Over time, you'll see patterns in what works best with almond flour, allowing you to refine your techniques.
   - *Confidence*: Documenting your successes boosts your confidence and motivates you to keep experimenting.
   - *Legacy*: Your journal becomes a personal recipe book filled with tried-and-true dishes and valuable insights.

Embrace the Adventure

Cooking with almond flour is an exciting journey filled with endless possibilities. By trying new recipes, connecting with like-minded individuals, and meticulously documenting your experiments, you'll continue to grow and innovate in the kitchen. Embrace the adventure, enjoy the process, and let your creativity shine.

By following these steps, you'll be well on your way to mastering the use of almond flour in your kitchen, enjoying its delicious taste, and reaping its numerous health benefits.

Conclusion

Congratulations on making it to the end of our Almond Flour Guide! Your dedication to learning about this versatile and nutritious ingredient is commendable. By now, you have delved into the myriad benefits of almond flour, discovered its versatility in the kitchen, and explored its suitability for various dietary needs. We're thrilled to have been part of your journey, and we hope you're excited to start experimenting with almond flour in your recipes.

Almond flour is a powerhouse ingredient that offers a wealth of nutritional benefits. Rich in protein, healthy fats, vitamins, and minerals, it serves as an excellent alternative to traditional flours. Whether you're looking to reduce your carbohydrate intake, manage gluten sensitivities, or simply enhance the nutritional profile of your meals, almond flour is a fantastic choice. Its high fiber content aids in digestion, while the abundance of vitamin E provides antioxidant properties that contribute to overall health.

One of the most remarkable aspects of almond flour is its versatility. You can use it in a wide range of recipes, from baked goods to savory dishes. It's perfect for making light and fluffy pancakes, deliciously moist muffins, or even crispy coatings for chicken and fish. The subtle, nutty flavor of almond flour adds a delightful twist to your culinary creations, elevating them to new heights.

As you start incorporating almond flour into your cooking, don't be afraid to experiment. Try substituting almond flour in your favorite recipes and see how it transforms the taste and texture. You might find that your go-to banana bread becomes even more decadent, or that your morning smoothies achieve a richer, creamier consistency with a spoonful of almond flour. The possibilities are endless, and the results can be truly rewarding.

When it comes to buying almond flour, quality matters. Look for brands that offer finely ground almond flour, as this will ensure a smoother texture in your recipes. Opt for blanched almond flour, which has the skins removed, for a finer and lighter result. You can find almond flour in most grocery stores, health food stores, or online retailers. Buying in bulk can be a cost-effective option, especially if you plan to use it frequently.

Proper storage of almond flour is essential to maintaining its freshness and quality. Store it in an airtight container in a cool, dark place, such as your pantry or refrigerator. Almond flour has a high oil content, so it can go rancid if exposed to heat, light, or air for extended periods. By taking these simple precautions, you can ensure that your almond flour remains fresh and ready to use whenever you need it.

As you embark on your almond flour journey, remember that patience and practice are key. Like any new ingredient, there may be a learning curve as you get accustomed to its unique properties. But don't let that discourage you. The more you experiment with almond flour, the more confident and creative you'll become. Soon enough, you'll be whipping up almond flour-based dishes with ease and impressing your family and friends with your culinary skills.

We encourage you to share your almond flour creations with others. Whether it's through social media, a food blog, or simply during family gatherings, sharing your experiences can inspire others to explore the wonders of almond flour. You might even exchange recipes and tips, further enriching your culinary repertoire.

In closing, we want to thank you for taking the time to complete this guide. Your commitment to enhancing your cooking skills and embracing healthier ingredients is truly inspiring. Almond flour is more than just an alternative to traditional flours; it's a gateway to a world of nutritious and delicious possibilities. By incorporating almond flour into your diet, you're making a positive choice for your health and well-being.

FAQs

What are the nutritional benefits of almond flour?

Almond flour is rich in protein, healthy fats, vitamins, and minerals. It provides a good source of fiber, aiding in digestion, and is packed with vitamin E, which offers antioxidant properties that contribute to overall health. Its low carbohydrate content makes it an excellent choice for those following low-carb or ketogenic diets.

How can I use almond flour in my recipes?

Almond flour is incredibly versatile and can be used in both sweet and savory recipes. It works well in baked goods like muffins, cookies, and pancakes, adding a moist and fluffy texture. You can also use it as a coating for meats like chicken or fish, or incorporate it into smoothies for extra creaminess.

Is almond flour suitable for gluten-free diets?

Yes, almond flour is naturally gluten-free, making it a great option for those with gluten sensitivities or celiac disease. It can be used as a direct substitute for wheat flour in many recipes, although it may require some adjustments in liquid amounts and baking times.

How should I store almond flour to keep it fresh?

To maintain the freshness and quality of almond flour, store it in an airtight container in a cool, dark place such as your pantry or refrigerator. Due to its high oil content, it can go rancid if exposed to heat, light, or air for prolonged periods. Following these storage tips will help keep your almond flour fresh and ready for use.

Can I substitute almond flour for regular flour in any recipe?

While almond flour can be substituted for regular flour in many recipes, there are some differences to consider. Almond flour is denser and absorbs more moisture, so you may need to adjust the liquid ingredients in your recipe. It also doesn't bind as well as gluten-containing flours, so adding an extra egg or a binding agent like xanthan gum can help achieve the desired texture.

Where can I buy high-quality almond flour?

You can find almond flour in most grocery stores, health food stores, or online retailers. Look for brands that offer finely ground, blanched almond flour for the best texture in your recipes. Buying in bulk can also be a cost-effective option if you plan to use it frequently.

What are some tips for baking with almond flour?

When baking with almond flour, it's important to remember that it browns faster than regular flour, so you may need to lower your oven temperature slightly. Also, because it lacks gluten, recipes may turn out denser. To counter this, you can combine almond flour with other gluten-free flour or add a binding agent like eggs. Experimenting and adjusting as needed will help you achieve the best results in your almond flour-based dishes.

References and Helpful Links

Dev, C. (2024, July 8). A guide to almond flour - LesserEvil. LesserEvil. https://lesserevil.com/blogs/health-wellness/a-guide-to-almond-flour/#:~:text=All%20you%20need%20are%20blanched,almond%20butter%20rather%20than%20flour.

Watson, M. (2021, August 4). Everything you need to know about almond flour. The Spruce Eats. https://www.thespruceeats.com/almond-flour-guide-4171541

WebMD Editorial Contributor. (2022, September 1). Health benefits of almond flour. WebMD. https://www.webmd.com/diet/health-benefits-almond-flour#:~:text=Almond%20flour%20is%20rich%20in,than%20women%20who%20do%20not.&text=Almond%20flour%20is%20a%20low%20glycemic%20index%20food.

Almond flour Nutrition, benefits, how to use and side effects - Dr. Axe. (2023, December 18). Dr. Axe. https://draxe.com/nutrition/almond-flour/

Sanford, A. (2023, April 8). 20+ "Foolproof" Almond Flour Recipes for Beginners. Foolproof Living. https://foolproofliving.com/almond-flour-recipes/

Almond Flour & Almond Meal | Recipes & Trends | Almond Basics. (n.d.).

https://www.almonds.com/why-almonds/recipes-and-trends/almond-basics/almond-flour

Rd, R. R. M. (2017, April 25). Why almond flour is better than most other flours. Healthline.
https://www.healthline.com/nutrition/almond-flour#:~:text=What%20Is%20Almond%20Flour%3F,names%20are%20sometimes%20used%20interchangeably.

www.ingramcontent.com/pod-product-compliance
Lightning Source LLC
LaVergne TN
LVHW010402070526
838199LV00065B/5875